OVERCOMING OCD FOR A LIFE OF BALANCE:

From Chaos to Clarity

BY

KATHERINE A. PENDLETON

Table of contents

Introduction

1. Understanding OCD: An Overview

    1.1 Defining OCD

    1.2 Common Types of OCD

    1.3 Causes and Risk Factors

2. Recognizing OCD Symptoms

    2.1 Obsessions: Intrusive Thoughts and Fears

    2.2 Compulsions: Repetitive Behaviors and Rituals

    2.3 Impact on Daily Life

3. Seeking Professional Help

    3.1 The Role of Mental Health Professionals

    3.2 Diagnosing OCD: Assessments and Evaluations

    3.3 Treatment Options: Therapy and Medication

4. Cognitive Behavioral Therapy (CBT)

    4.1 Understanding CBT and Its Effectiveness for OCD

4.2 Exposure and Response Prevention (ERP)

4.3 Cognitive Restructuring

5. Mindfulness and Relaxation Techniques

5.1 Introduction to Mindfulness

5.2 Mindfulness-Based Stress Reduction (MBSR)

5.3 Deep Breathing and Progressive Muscle Relaxation

6. Building Healthy Habits and Routines

6.1 Establishing Structure and Organization

6.2 Prioritizing Self-Care

6.3 Healthy Sleep Habits

7. Managing Stress and Anxiety

7.1 Stress-Reduction Techniques

7.2 Anxiety Management Strategies

7.3 Coping with Uncertainty

8. Enhancing Relationships and Social Support

8.1 Communicating with Loved Ones about OCD

8.2 Building a Support Network

8.3 Balancing Independence and Interdependence

9. Maintaining Long-Term Recovery

9.1 Relapse Prevention Strategies

9.2 Self-Reflection and Self-Care Practices

9.3 Continuing Professional Support

Conclusion

Introduction

Welcome to the world of "Overcoming OCD for a Life of Balance:From Chaos to Clarity" This book is a comprehensive guide designed to support individuals who are facing the challenges of obsessive-compulsive disorder (OCD) and seeking a balanced and fulfilling life. Whether you are personally affected by OCD or you are supporting someone who is, this book aims to provide you with knowledge, strategies, and insights to navigate the complexities of OCD and move towards a life of greater harmony.

OCD is a mental health condition characterized by intrusive thoughts, fears, and repetitive behaviors or rituals. It can significantly impact daily life, relationships, and overall well-being. However, with the right understanding, tools, and support, it is possible to manage OCD effectively and regain control over your life.

In this book, we will delve into various aspects of OCD, starting with an exploration of its common types, causes, and risk factors. We will then examine the nature of obsessions and how they manifest as intrusive thoughts and fears, as well as the compulsions that drive repetitive behaviors and rituals. Understanding the impact of OCD on daily life is crucial for developing effective coping strategies and creating a life of balance.

Professional support plays a vital role in overcoming OCD, so we will discuss the importance of mental health professionals in diagnosing OCD and conducting assessments and evaluations. Treatment options, including therapy and medication, will be explored in detail, providing you with a comprehensive understanding of the available interventions.

Cognitive Behavioral Therapy (CBT), Exposure and Response Prevention (ERP), and other evidence-based treatment approaches will be examined, along with mindfulness-based practices and stress reduction techniques that can enhance your overall well-being. We will also explore self-reflection and self-care practices, establishing structure and organization, and building a support network to create a solid foundation for your journey towards balance and recovery.

Throughout this book, you will find practical tips, exercises, and examples to help you apply the concepts and strategies discussed. It is important to remember that everyone's journey with OCD is unique, and what works for one person may not work for another. However, by utilizing the knowledge and tools provided in this book, you will be equipped with a wide range of resources to tailor your own path towards overcoming OCD and living a more balanced, fulfilling life.

Now, let's embark on this transformative journey together, where you will gain insights, develop skills, and discover the resilience and strength within you to overcome OCD and embrace a life of balance.

CHAPTER 1

1.1. Defining OCD

OCD stands for Obsessive-Compulsive Disorder. It is a mental health disorder characterized by recurring, intrusive thoughts (obsessions) and repetitive behaviors or mental acts (compulsions) that individuals feel compelled to perform. These obsessions and compulsions often cause distress and can significantly interfere with daily functioning and quality of life.

Obsessions are unwanted and distressing thoughts, images, or urges that repeatedly intrude upon a person's mind. Common obsessions may revolve around themes like cleanliness, symmetry, harm, or contamination. Examples of obsessions include an intense fear of germs, an excessive need for order or symmetry, or distressing thoughts of causing harm to oneself or others.

Compulsions are repetitive behaviors or mental acts that individuals feel driven to perform in response to their obsessions. These behaviors are typically aimed at reducing anxiety or preventing perceived harm. Examples of compulsions include excessive hand washing, repeated checking of locks or appliances, counting or arranging objects in a particular order, or seeking reassurance repeatedly.

It's important to note that OCD is a chronic condition, and while the specific symptoms may vary among individuals, the underlying features are the presence of obsessions and compulsions that cause distress and significantly impact daily life. Treatment, including therapy and medication, can be effective in managing and reducing the symptoms of OCD, allowing individuals to lead more balanced and fulfilling lives.

1.2 Common types of OCD

There are several common types of OCD, each characterized by specific themes or patterns of obsessions and compulsions. Here are a few examples:

1.Contamination OCD: This type of OCD involves an intense fear of contamination or germs. Individuals may excessively wash their hands, avoid touching certain objects or surfaces, or engage in cleaning rituals to alleviate their anxiety.

2. Checking OCD: People with OCD have a persistent fear of harm or danger and feel compelled to check things repeatedly. This could involve repeatedly checking locks, appliances, or personal belongings to ensure they are secure or in the right order.

3. Symmetry and Ordering OCD: This subtype is characterized by an overwhelming need for symmetry, exactness, or orderliness. Individuals with

this type of OCD may spend excessive amounts of time arranging objects, aligning items perfectly, or feeling distressed when things are not symmetrical.

4. Hoarding OCD: Hoarding involves an excessive accumulation of possessions and an inability to discard them, resulting in significant clutter and difficulty maintaining living spaces. People with hoarding OCD often feel extreme distress when attempting to throw away items, leading to severe clutter and an inability to function in their living environments.

5. Intrusive Thoughts OCD: This subtype involves intrusive and distressing thoughts or mental images that go against an individual's values or beliefs. These thoughts may be violent, sexual, or blasphemous in nature and can cause significant anxiety and distress.

6. Just-Right OCD: Just-right OCD is characterized by a persistent feeling of things being "just right" or a need for a specific order or positioning. Individuals may repeatedly perform certain actions until they feel a sense of completeness or satisfaction.

It's important to note that these are just a few examples, and OCD symptoms can vary widely among individuals. Some people may experience a combination of different OCD subtypes, and symptoms can change over time. Seeking professional help from a mental health professional experienced in treating OCD is crucial for accurate diagnosis and effective treatment.

1.3. Causes and risk factors

The exact causes of OCD are not yet fully understood. However, research suggests that a combination of genetic, neurobiological, and environmental factors contribute to the development of the disorder. Here are some potential causes and risk factors associated with OCD:

1. Genetic Factors: There is evidence to suggest that OCD can run in families, indicating a genetic component. People with a family history of OCD may be at a higher risk of developing the disorder.

2. Neurobiological Factors: Studies have shown that abnormalities in certain brain structures and neurotransmitter imbalances, such as serotonin, dopamine, and glutamate, may play a role in the development of OCD. These neurobiological factors can impact the functioning of brain circuits involved in regulating thoughts and behaviors.

3. Environmental Factors: Certain environmental factors may contribute to the development or exacerbation of OCD. These can include:

Childhood Trauma: Some studies have found a link between early life trauma, such as physical or sexual abuse, and the development of OCD later in life.

Stressful Life Events: Major life events, such as significant loss, changes, or traumatic experiences, can trigger or worsen OCD symptoms.

Learned Behaviors: Observing or experiencing behaviors associated with OCD in family members or peers can influence the development of similar patterns of thoughts and actions.

4. Cognitive Factors: Some individuals with OCD may have specific cognitive tendencies that contribute to the disorder. This includes having an inflated sense of responsibility, perfectionistic tendencies, or a tendency to overestimate potential threats or dangers.

5. Personality Factors: Certain personality traits, such as high levels of anxiety, perfectionism, or a tendency towards rigidity and orderliness, may increase the risk of developing OCD.

It's important to note that while these factors may increase the likelihood of developing OCD, they do not guarantee the development of the disorder. OCD is a complex condition, and individual experiences can vary greatly. Seeking professional help from a mental health provider is crucial for a comprehensive evaluation and understanding of the specific factors contributing to an individual's OCD symptoms.

CHAPTER 2

2.1 Obsessions: Intrusive Thoughts and Fears

Obsessions are intrusive and distressing thoughts, images, or urges that repeatedly come to mind and cause significant anxiety or distress. They are one of the core features of OCD. Here are some common types of obsessions:

1. Contamination Obsessions: These involve fears of being contaminated by germs, dirt, or harmful substances. Individuals may worry excessively about coming into contact with contaminants and may engage in rituals like excessive hand washing or avoiding certain places to reduce their anxiety.

2. Fear of Harming Self or Others: Some people with OCD have intrusive thoughts or fears of causing harm to themselves or others. These thoughts may involve images

of violent or aggressive acts and can be distressing. Individuals may engage in compulsions to prevent harm or seek reassurance from others.

3. Symmetry and Orderliness Obsessions: These obsessions involve an intense need for things to be symmetrical, aligned, or in perfect order. Individuals may have distressing thoughts when things are not arranged correctly and may spend excessive time and energy organizing and arranging objects.

4. Unwanted Sexual or Taboo Thoughts: Some individuals with OCD experience intrusive thoughts of a sexual nature or thoughts that go against their personal values or beliefs. These thoughts can be distressing and cause significant anxiety and guilt.

5. Religious or Moral Obsessions: These obsessions involve excessive concerns about

religious or moral matters. Individuals may have intrusive thoughts that go against their religious beliefs or fear that they have committed immoral acts, leading to distress and a need to seek reassurance or engage in compulsive behaviors.

6. Health and Illness Obsessions: Individuals with health-related obsessions may constantly worry about having a serious illness or medical condition. They may excessively research symptoms, seek medical reassurance, or repeatedly visit doctors to alleviate their fears.

It's important to remember that these obsessions are distressing and unwanted, and individuals with OCD often recognize that their thoughts are irrational. However, attempts to suppress or ignore these obsessions often lead to increased anxiety. Treatment, including therapy and medication, can help individuals manage and reduce the impact of these obsessions on their daily lives.

2.2 Compulsions: Repetitive Behaviors and Rituals

Compulsions are repetitive behaviors or mental acts that individuals with OCD feel compelled to perform in response to their obsessions. These compulsions are aimed at reducing anxiety, preventing harm, or neutralizing obsessive thoughts. Here are some common types of compulsions:

1. Cleaning and Washing Rituals: Individuals with contamination obsessions often engage in excessive cleaning and washing behaviors. They may spend excessive time and effort cleaning themselves, their surroundings, or specific objects to alleviate their fears of contamination.

2. Checking Behaviors: Checking compulsions involve repeatedly checking

things to ensure safety, prevent harm, or ease anxiety. This can include checking locks, appliances, or personal belongings, such as doors, stoves, or bags, even when there is no logical reason to do so.

3. Ordering and Arranging Rituals: People with a need for symmetry or orderliness may engage in compulsive behaviors related to arranging objects or performing tasks in a particular sequence. They may spend excessive time aligning items, organizing possessions, or following rigid routines to achieve a sense of order and relief.

4. Repeating Actions: Repeating compulsions involve performing actions or rituals multiple times until they feel "just right" or a sense of completeness is achieved. This can include actions like going in and out of a doorway, repeating words or phrases, or redoing tasks multiple times.

5. Mental Rituals: Some compulsions are performed mentally rather than physically. Individuals may engage in repetitive mental rituals, such as counting, reciting specific phrases or prayers, or mentally reviewing past events, in an attempt to neutralize obsessions or prevent harm.

6. Seeking Reassurance: Individuals with OCD often seek reassurance from others to alleviate their anxiety. They may repeatedly ask for reassurance or seek confirmation that their fears are unfounded. However, this seeking of reassurance can become a compulsive behavior in itself.

It's important to note that compulsions are meant to provide temporary relief from anxiety but can reinforce the cycle of obsessions and compulsions in the long run. Treatment, such as cognitive-behavioral therapy (CBT) with a focus on exposure and response prevention (ERP), can help individuals reduce and manage their compulsions and break free from the cycle of OCD.

2.3 Impact on daily life

OCD can have a significant impact on various aspects of a person's daily life. The obsessions and compulsions associated with OCD can consume a significant amount of time, energy, and mental focus, affecting an individual's functioning and overall well-being. Here are some ways OCD can impact daily life:

1. Interference with Daily Activities: OCD can interfere with routine activities, such as getting ready in the morning, going to work or school, or completing household tasks. The time-consuming nature of obsessions and compulsions can disrupt daily schedules and make it difficult to meet responsibilities and obligations.

2. Impaired Social Relationships: OCD can strain relationships with family, friends, and

romantic partners. The preoccupation with obsessions and the need to perform compulsions can lead to social withdrawal, avoidance of social situations, and difficulty engaging in activities or events that others may enjoy.

3. Occupational Challenges: OCD symptoms can affect work or academic performance. The need to engage in rituals or repetitive behaviors may result in decreased productivity, difficulty meeting deadlines, or challenges in maintaining focus and concentration.

4. Emotional Distress: Living with OCD can cause significant emotional distress. The intrusive thoughts, fears, and the constant need to perform compulsions can lead to high levels of anxiety, guilt, shame, and frustration. This emotional burden can impact mood, self-esteem, and overall quality of life.

5. Physical Toll: The repetitive behaviors associated with OCD, such as excessive hand washing or checking, can take a physical toll on the body. For example, frequent hand washing may lead to dry or irritated skin, and repetitive checking behaviors can cause physical fatigue and strain.

6. Financial Impact: In some cases, the financial burden of OCD treatment, including therapy and medications, can impact individuals and their families. The costs associated with seeking professional help and managing the condition can add stress to an already challenging situation.

It's important to recognize the significant impact OCD can have on daily life and seek appropriate treatment and support. With proper management and intervention, individuals can learn to cope with their symptoms, reduce their impact, and regain a sense of balance and well-being.

CHAPTER 3

3.1 Role of mental health professionals

Mental health professionals play a crucial role in the assessment, diagnosis, and treatment of OCD. They are trained to provide the necessary support and interventions to individuals experiencing OCD symptoms. Here are some key roles mental health professionals play in helping individuals with OCD:

1. Assessment and Diagnosis: Mental health professionals, such as psychologists or psychiatrists, conduct comprehensive assessments to evaluate and diagnose OCD. They gather information about the individual's symptoms, history, and functioning to make an accurate diagnosis.

2. Treatment Planning: Mental health professionals work with individuals to develop personalized treatment plans based

on their specific needs and goals. They consider various factors, such as the severity of symptoms, individual strengths, and available resources, to create an effective treatment strategy.

3. Therapy: Therapies, particularly cognitive-behavioral therapy (CBT), are considered the first-line treatment for OCD. Mental health professionals provide CBT, including specialized techniques such as Exposure and Response Prevention (ERP). ERP helps individuals confront their fears and gradually reduce their reliance on compulsive behaviors.

4. Medication Management: In some cases, mental health professionals, usually psychiatrists, may prescribe medication to complement therapy. Selective serotonin reuptake inhibitors (SSRIs) are often prescribed as a first-line medication for OCD. Mental health professionals monitor

medication effectiveness, adjust dosages, and manage potential side effects.

5. Education and Psychoeducation: Mental health professionals educate individuals and their families about OCD, its causes, and available treatments. They help individuals understand the nature of OCD, challenge misconceptions, and provide psychoeducation on strategies for managing symptoms and improving overall well-being.

6. Support and Empowerment: Mental health professionals offer support, empathy, and guidance throughout the treatment process. They provide a safe and non-judgmental space for individuals to express their concerns, fears, and challenges associated with OCD. Mental health professionals empower individuals by teaching coping skills, problem-solving techniques, and resilience-building strategies.

7. Relapse Prevention: Mental health professionals assist individuals in developing relapse prevention strategies to maintain progress and manage potential setbacks. They help individuals identify triggers, develop coping mechanisms, and establish long-term strategies for managing OCD symptoms.

Remember, the specific roles and expertise of mental health professionals may vary depending on their training, specialization, and professional background. Seeking help from qualified professionals experienced in treating OCD is essential for effective management and recovery.

3.2. Diagnosing OCD: Assessments and Evaluations

Diagnosing OCD typically involves a comprehensive assessment and evaluation process conducted by mental health professionals. Here are some common methods used in the diagnostic process:

1. Clinical Interviews: Mental health professionals conduct clinical interviews to gather detailed information about an individual's symptoms, experiences, and history. These interviews help assess the presence of obsessions and compulsions, their impact on daily functioning, and any associated distress or impairment.

2. Diagnostic Criteria: Mental health professionals refer to diagnostic criteria outlined in the Diagnostic and Statistical Manual of Mental Disorders (DSM-5), which provides a standardized set of criteria for diagnosing mental health conditions, including OCD. The DSM-5 criteria for OCD specify the presence of obsessions and/or compulsions that are time-consuming, cause significant distress, and interfere with daily life.

3. Symptom Assessment Tools: Mental health professionals may use self-report

questionnaires or structured interviews that assess the specific symptoms and severity of OCD. These assessment tools can help quantify the frequency, intensity, and impact of obsessions and compulsions, aiding in the diagnostic process and treatment planning.

4. Differential Diagnosis: Mental health professionals differentiate OCD from other mental health conditions that may share similar symptoms. This is important to ensure an accurate diagnosis and appropriate treatment. Conditions that may be considered in the differential diagnosis include other anxiety disorders, body dysmorphic disorder, and hoarding disorder.

5. Medical Evaluation: In some cases, mental health professionals may recommend a medical evaluation to rule out any underlying medical conditions that could be contributing to or exacerbating

OCD symptoms. Certain medical conditions, such as infections or neurological disorders, can present with symptoms similar to OCD.

6. Collaboration and Consultation: Mental health professionals may collaborate with other healthcare providers, such as psychiatrists or primary care physicians, to gather additional information, review medical history, and discuss treatment options. Collaboration ensures a comprehensive assessment and holistic approach to treatment.

The assessment and evaluation process aims to gather detailed information, understand the individual's experiences and symptoms, and make an accurate diagnosis. This diagnostic process helps inform treatment planning, as it guides the selection of appropriate therapeutic interventions and interventions tailored to the individual's specific needs.

3.3 Treatment Options: Therapy and Medication

Treatment for OCD typically involves a combination of therapy and, in some cases, medication. Here are the main treatment options for OCD:

1. Cognitive-Behavioral Therapy (CBT): CBT is the most effective form of psychotherapy for OCD. Specifically, a subtype of CBT called Exposure and Response Prevention (ERP) is often used. ERP involves gradually exposing individuals to situations or thoughts that trigger their obsessions while preventing the corresponding compulsive behaviors or rituals. This process helps individuals learn to tolerate the anxiety caused by obsessions without resorting to compulsions. CBT also includes other techniques, such as cognitive restructuring, which involves challenging and modifying unhelpful beliefs and thought patterns related to OCD.

2. Medication: Selective serotonin reuptake inhibitors (SSRIs) are commonly prescribed as the first-line medication treatment for OCD. SSRIs increase the levels of serotonin, a neurotransmitter in the brain that regulates mood and anxiety. These medications can help reduce the severity of OCD symptoms. Examples of SSRIs commonly used for OCD include fluoxetine, fluvoxamine, sertraline, and escitalopram. It's important to consult with a psychiatrist or medical professional for medication assessment, prescription, and management.

3. Combination Therapy: In some cases, a combination of CBT and medication may be recommended for individuals with OCD, particularly when symptoms are severe or have not responded adequately to either treatment alone. CBT and medication can complement each other, with CBT addressing the underlying thought patterns and behaviors and medication helping to alleviate symptoms and reduce anxiety.

4. Support Groups: Support groups, either in-person or online, can be valuable for individuals with OCD. These groups provide a supportive environment where individuals can share their experiences, gain insights from others who have similar challenges, and receive encouragement and understanding. Support groups can also offer practical tips and strategies for managing OCD symptoms.

5. Family Therapy: Involving family members in the treatment process can be beneficial, especially when OCD affects family dynamics and relationships. Family therapy can help educate family members about OCD, improve communication and support within the family, and assist in reducing accommodation behaviors that inadvertently reinforce the OCD symptoms.

6. Self-Help Strategies: Self-help strategies, such as self-education about OCD,

practicing stress management techniques, engaging in regular exercise, and maintaining a healthy lifestyle, can be helpful in managing OCD symptoms. However, these strategies are typically most effective when combined with professional treatment.

The choice of treatment approach depends on the individual's preferences, the severity of symptoms, and their response to previous treatments. It's important to work with qualified mental health professionals who specialize in OCD treatment to develop an individualized treatment plan and receive ongoing support.

In addition to cognitive-behavioral therapy (CBT) and medication, there are several other treatment options that can be considered for OCD. While the effectiveness of these treatments may vary for each individual, they can complement traditional therapy approaches. Some additional treatment options for OCD include:

1. Acceptance and Commitment Therapy (ACT): ACT is a form of psychotherapy that focuses on accepting unwanted thoughts and feelings while committing to actions that align with personal values. ACT can help individuals develop psychological flexibility and reduce the impact of OCD on their lives. It involves mindfulness techniques, cognitive defusion exercises, and value-based goal setting.

2. Dialectical Behavior Therapy (DBT): DBT combines elements of CBT with mindfulness and acceptance strategies. Originally developed to treat borderline personality disorder, DBT has also shown effectiveness in addressing OCD symptoms. It emphasizes skills training in emotional regulation, distress tolerance, interpersonal effectiveness, and mindfulness.

3. Psychodynamic Therapy: Psychodynamic therapy explores the underlying psychological processes, past experiences, and unconscious conflicts that may contribute to OCD symptoms. It aims to increase self-awareness and insight into the roots of obsessions and compulsions, facilitating long-term psychological growth and symptom reduction.

4. Group Therapy: Group therapy brings together individuals with OCD to share experiences, offer support, and learn from one another. Group therapy can provide a sense of belonging, reduce feelings of isolation, and offer a supportive environment for practicing new coping strategies. It may be conducted alongside individual therapy or as a standalone treatment.

5. Virtual Reality Exposure Therapy (VRET): VRET involves exposing individuals to virtual environments that

simulate situations triggering their OCD symptoms. This immersive therapy allows individuals to gradually confront their fears and obsessions in a controlled setting, helping them learn to tolerate anxiety and reduce avoidance behaviors.

6. Transcranial Magnetic Stimulation (TMS): TMS is a non-invasive procedure that uses magnetic fields to stimulate specific areas of the brain. It has shown promise as a potential treatment for OCD, particularly for individuals who have not responded well to other interventions. TMS is typically administered under the guidance of a psychiatrist or neurologist.

7. Deep Brain Stimulation (DBS): DBS is a surgical procedure that involves implanting electrodes in specific areas of the brain to modulate neural activity. It is considered a treatment option for severe and treatment-resistant OCD. DBS requires careful evaluation and is typically reserved

for individuals who have not responded to other therapies.

It's important to note that not all treatment options may be suitable or readily accessible for everyone. The choice of treatment should be based on a thorough evaluation by a qualified mental health professional and tailored to the individual's specific needs, preferences, and treatment response.

CHAPTER 4

4.1 Understanding CBT and Its Effectiveness for OCD

Cognitive-Behavioral Therapy (CBT) is a widely recognized and effective treatment approach for OCD. It is a structured and goal-oriented form of psychotherapy that focuses on identifying and modifying unhelpful thoughts, beliefs, and behaviors associated with OCD. Here's a breakdown of CBT and its effectiveness for OCD:

1. Cognitive Restructuring: CBT for OCD involves identifying and challenging negative and distorted thoughts related to obsessions. It helps individuals recognize that their thoughts are not accurate reflections of reality and assists in replacing them with more realistic and adaptive beliefs. By restructuring cognitions, individuals can reduce the anxiety and distress triggered by obsessions.

2. Exposure and Response Prevention (ERP): ERP is a core component of CBT for OCD and involves deliberately exposing individuals to situations, thoughts, or objects that trigger their obsessions. The goal is to confront the fears and anxiety associated with the obsessions without resorting to the accompanying compulsive behaviors or rituals. Over time, repeated exposure without engaging in the compulsions helps individuals learn that their feared outcomes are unlikely to occur, reducing the intensity of obsessions.

3. Skills Development: CBT equips individuals with specific skills and strategies to manage OCD symptoms. These skills may include relaxation techniques, mindfulness exercises, thought-stopping techniques, and problem-solving strategies. By learning and practicing these skills, individuals develop a toolbox of coping mechanisms to effectively manage their symptoms and reduce the impact of OCD on their lives.

4. Homework Assignments: CBT often involves assigning homework between therapy sessions. These assignments may include exposure exercises, practicing new coping strategies, or tracking and challenging obsessive thoughts. Homework assignments help individuals reinforce the skills learned in therapy and generalize them to real-life situations.

Effectiveness of CBT for OCD:

CBT, particularly ERP, has been extensively studied and proven to be highly effective in reducing OCD symptoms. Research studies consistently demonstrate that the majority of individuals with OCD show significant improvement with CBT, and many experience a substantial reduction in symptom severity.

CBT for OCD has several advantages:

1. Long-Term Benefits: CBT focuses on addressing the underlying thoughts and behaviors associated with OCD, leading to lasting improvements even after therapy has ended.

2. Reduction in Relapse: CBT, especially ERP, emphasizes developing skills to manage symptoms independently, reducing the likelihood of relapse.

3. Customized Treatment: CBT is tailored to the individual's specific OCD symptoms and their unique triggers, allowing for personalized treatment plans.

4. Empowerment and Independence: CBT empowers individuals to take an active role in managing their symptoms, providing them with skills and strategies they can use throughout their lives.

It's important to note that CBT for OCD is typically conducted by trained mental health professionals, such as psychologists or therapists, who specialize in the treatment of OCD. The effectiveness of CBT may vary for each individual, and the duration of treatment can range from several weeks to several months, depending on the severity of symptoms and individual progress.

4.2 Exposure and Response Prevention (ERP)

Exposure and Response Prevention (ERP) is a key component of cognitive-behavioral therapy (CBT) and is considered the most effective treatment approach for obsessive-compulsive disorder (OCD). ERP involves systematically exposing individuals to situations, thoughts, or objects that trigger their obsessions, while simultaneously preventing the corresponding compulsive behaviors or rituals. The goal of ERP is to help individuals learn to tolerate the anxiety caused by obsessions without resorting to compulsions, ultimately reducing the intensity and frequency of OCD symptoms.

Here's how ERP typically works:

1. Creating an Exposure Hierarchy: With the guidance of a mental health professional, individuals work together to create an exposure hierarchy. This hierarchy is a list of situations or triggers that elicit obsessive thoughts or anxiety, ranked from least distressing to most distressing. It helps individuals gradually confront their fears in a systematic manner.

2. Exposure Sessions: In exposure sessions, individuals are exposed to the situations or triggers identified in the hierarchy. The exposure can be in the form of real-life situations or through imaginal exposure (imagining the feared scenarios). The exposure is carried out without engaging in the accompanying compulsive behaviors or

rituals that typically provide temporary relief.

3. Response Prevention: During the exposure sessions, individuals are actively discouraged from engaging in the usual compulsions or rituals. This is the "response prevention" aspect of ERP. By resisting the urge to perform compulsions, individuals have an opportunity to learn that their feared outcomes are unlikely to occur and that their anxiety gradually diminishes over time.

4. Gradual Progression: ERP is typically conducted in a gradual and systematic manner. Individuals start with exposures that evoke mild to moderate anxiety and gradually progress to more challenging situations as they build tolerance and gain confidence. This step-by-step approach ensures that individuals do not feel overwhelmed and allows for steady progress.

5. Habituation and Learning: Through repeated exposure to feared situations without engaging in compulsive behaviors, individuals experience habituation, meaning that their anxiety naturally decreases over time. This process helps them learn that their fears are unfounded and that they can tolerate the discomfort associated with their obsessions.

6. Generalization and Maintenance: The skills learned during ERP sessions are then applied to real-life situations outside of therapy. Individuals are encouraged to continue practicing exposure exercises independently to maintain progress and prevent relapse.

ERP is highly effective because it directly targets the core mechanisms that maintain OCD symptoms. It helps individuals confront their fears, reduce avoidance behaviors, and gradually retrain their brain to respond differently to obsessions. ERP is typically conducted under the guidance of a trained mental health professional who provides support, guidance, and feedback throughout the treatment process.

It's important to note that ERP can initially cause increased anxiety and discomfort as individuals confront their fears. However, with time and practice, the anxiety diminishes, and individuals experience significant symptom reduction and improved quality of life.

4.3 Cognitive Restructuring

Cognitive restructuring is a cognitive-behavioral technique commonly used in the treatment of various mental health conditions, including obsessive-compulsive disorder (OCD). It involves identifying and challenging unhelpful or distorted thoughts and beliefs that contribute to distressing emotions and behaviors. By modifying these cognitive patterns, individuals can develop a more realistic and adaptive perspective, leading to improved emotional well-being and behavior change.

Here's an overview of the process of cognitive restructuring:

1. Identifying Automatic Thoughts: Automatic thoughts are the rapid, unconscious thoughts that pop into our minds in response to specific situations or triggers. In the context of OCD, these automatic thoughts are often negative, distorted, and exaggerated, fueling anxiety, guilt, or a sense of impending danger. Cognitive restructuring begins by recognizing and capturing these automatic thoughts.

2. Evaluating the Evidence: Once automatic thoughts are identified, the next step is to evaluate the evidence supporting or contradicting these thoughts. This involves

examining the facts objectively and challenging the accuracy of the thoughts. Individuals are encouraged to ask themselves questions like, "What evidence supports this thought?" and "Is there any evidence against this thought?"

3. Examining Cognitive Distortions: Cognitive distortions are biased and irrational thinking patterns that contribute to negative thoughts and emotions. Examples of common cognitive distortions in OCD include catastrophic thinking, black-and-white thinking, overgeneralization, and personalization. By identifying these distortions, individuals can recognize when their thoughts may be distorted and not based on reality.

4. Generating Alternative Thoughts: In cognitive restructuring, individuals work to generate alternative, more balanced, and rational thoughts that counteract the initial automatic thoughts. This step involves

brainstorming alternative explanations or perspectives that are more realistic and less anxiety-provoking. The aim is to develop thoughts that are more helpful, accurate, and aligned with evidence.

5. Replacing Thoughts and Practice: Once alternative thoughts are identified, individuals are encouraged to actively replace their automatic thoughts with these more adaptive thoughts. This may involve mentally rehearsing the new thoughts or using positive affirmations. Repeated practice and reinforcement help individuals strengthen the new cognitive patterns and make them more automatic.

6. Behavioral Integration: Cognitive restructuring is often combined with behavioral strategies to reinforce the new cognitive patterns. As individuals challenge and modify their thoughts, they can also engage in behaviors that align with their new perspectives. This integration between

cognition and behavior helps individuals solidify the changes and maintain progress.

Cognitive restructuring is a collaborative process between the individual and a mental health professional, such as a therapist or psychologist. The professional provides guidance, support, and feedback throughout the process, helping individuals identify and challenge their unhelpful thoughts effectively.

By modifying cognitive patterns and developing a more balanced perspective, individuals with OCD can reduce distress, anxiety, and the frequency and intensity of obsessive thoughts. Cognitive restructuring is an essential component of cognitive-behavioral therapy (CBT) and can greatly contribute to the overall treatment of OCD.

CHAPTER 5

5.1 Introduction to Mindfulness

Mindfulness is a practice and state of mind that involves paying intentional attention to the present moment, without judgment or attachment. It is derived from ancient Buddhist traditions but has gained significant popularity and recognition in contemporary psychology and wellness practices. Mindfulness involves cultivating a non-reactive awareness of one's thoughts, feelings, bodily sensations, and the surrounding environment.

Here's an introduction to mindfulness and its key principles:

1. Present-Moment Awareness: Mindfulness emphasizes bringing one's attention to the present moment, rather than dwelling on the past or worrying about the future. It involves observing one's experiences as they

arise, without getting caught up in
judgments, interpretations, or distractions.

2. Non-Judgmental Acceptance:
Mindfulness involves accepting one's
present-moment experiences without
judgment. It means acknowledging
thoughts, emotions, and sensations as they
are, without labeling them as good or bad,
right or wrong. This non-judgmental stance
fosters self-compassion, curiosity, and
openness.

3. Focus on Sensations and Breath:
Mindfulness often involves directing
attention to the sensations of the body or
the breath. This anchoring in physical
sensations serves as an anchor to the
present moment and helps individuals stay
grounded in their experience. By focusing
on the breath or bodily sensations,
individuals cultivate a sense of calm and
centeredness.

4. Cultivating Observing Awareness: Mindfulness encourages the development of a curious and observant stance toward one's thoughts, emotions, and sensations. Rather than getting caught up in the content of these experiences, mindfulness involves noticing them as passing mental events, without getting entangled or overwhelmed by them.

5. Letting Go of Attachment: Mindfulness encourages letting go of attachment to thoughts, emotions, or external outcomes. It involves recognizing that thoughts and emotions are transient and do not define one's identity. By letting go of attachment, individuals can develop a greater sense of inner freedom and reduce the influence of automatic reactions.

6. Cultivating Compassion and Kindness: Mindfulness practice often includes elements of self-compassion and compassion for others. It involves

cultivating a kind and gentle attitude toward oneself and others, fostering a sense of empathy, understanding, and connection.

Benefits of Mindfulness:

Mindfulness practice has been associated with various physical, mental, and emotional benefits, including:

- Reduced stress, anxiety, and depression
- Improved attention, focus, and cognitive flexibility
- Enhanced emotional regulation and resilience
- Better self-awareness and self-compassion
- Improved relationships and communication
- Increased overall well-being and life satisfaction

Mindfulness can be cultivated through formal practices, such as seated meditation, body scans, or mindful movement (e.g., yoga), as well as informal practices, such as bringing mindful awareness to daily activities like eating, walking, or listening.

While mindfulness is accessible to everyone, it is often recommended to learn from experienced teachers or through structured mindfulness programs to deepen the practice and fully benefit from its transformative potential.

5.2 Mindfulness-Based Stress Reduction (MBSR)

Mindfulness-Based Stress Reduction (MBSR) is a structured program that combines mindfulness meditation, body awareness, and yoga to help individuals manage stress, cope with physical and emotional challenges, and enhance overall well-being. It was developed by Dr. Jon Kabat-Zinn in the late 1970s and is now widely recognized and implemented in various healthcare and therapeutic settings.

The MBSR program typically spans eight weeks and involves weekly group sessions, daily home practice, and guided meditation recordings. Here are some key components and principles of MBSR:

1. Mindfulness Meditation: The core practice in MBSR is mindfulness meditation, which involves intentionally paying attention to the present moment, non-judgmentally and with curiosity. Participants are guided through different meditation techniques, such as breath awareness, body scan, and loving-kindness meditation, to cultivate mindfulness skills.

2. Body Awareness: MBSR emphasizes developing a heightened awareness of bodily sensations, movements, and postures. Through practices like the body scan, gentle yoga, and mindful movement exercises, participants learn to observe physical sensations, release tension, and develop a

deeper connection between the mind and body.

3. Non-Judgmental Awareness: MBSR encourages cultivating a non-judgmental and accepting attitude toward one's experiences. Participants learn to observe thoughts, emotions, and sensations without labeling them as good or bad, right or wrong. This non-judgmental stance fosters self-compassion and reduces the tendency to react impulsively or negatively to challenging situations.

4. Coping with Stressors: MBSR teaches participants to respond more effectively to stressors and life challenges. By cultivating mindfulness, individuals develop the capacity to pause, observe their reactions, and choose more skillful responses instead of automatic and habitual reactions. This can lead to reduced stress, improved emotional regulation, and enhanced coping strategies.

5. Integration into Daily Life: MBSR emphasizes the integration of mindfulness into daily activities. Participants are encouraged to bring mindful awareness to routine tasks, such as eating, walking, and interacting with others. This helps extend the benefits of mindfulness beyond formal meditation practice and promotes a greater sense of presence and engagement in everyday life.

Research has shown that MBSR can be effective in reducing stress, anxiety, depression, and pain, as well as improving overall well-being. It has been applied in various settings, including healthcare, education, workplaces, and community programs.

It's important to note that MBSR is typically taught by qualified instructors who have undergone training in the program. Participating in an MBSR course provides structured guidance, group support, and the opportunity to learn and practice mindfulness in a safe and supportive environment.

5.3 Deep Breathing and Progressive Muscle Relaxation

Deep breathing and progressive muscle relaxation are relaxation techniques commonly used to reduce stress, promote relaxation, and manage anxiety. They can be practiced independently or as part of a broader stress management or mindfulness program. Here's an overview of each technique:

1. Deep Breathing:
Deep breathing, also known as diaphragmatic breathing or belly breathing, involves consciously taking slow, deep breaths to activate the body's relaxation response. Here's how to practice deep breathing:

- Find a comfortable position, either sitting or lying down.
- Place one hand on your abdomen, just below your ribcage.
- Take a slow, deep breath in through your nose, allowing your abdomen to rise as you fill your lungs with air.
- Exhale slowly through your mouth, letting your abdomen fall as you release the breath.
- Focus your attention on the sensation of the breath entering and leaving your body.
- Continue this deep breathing pattern for several minutes, allowing your body and mind to relax with each breath.

Deep breathing helps activate the body's parasympathetic nervous system, which promotes a sense of calm and relaxation. It can be practiced anytime, anywhere, and is particularly helpful during times of stress, anxiety, or when feeling overwhelmed.

2. Progressive Muscle Relaxation (PMR):

Progressive muscle relaxation is a technique that involves systematically tensing and then relaxing different muscle groups in the body. The aim is to release physical tension and promote a state of deep relaxation. Here's how to practice progressive muscle relaxation:

- Find a quiet and comfortable space where you can lie down or sit in a relaxed position.
- Begin by focusing on your breathing and taking a few deep breaths to center yourself.
- Start with a specific muscle group, such as your hands or feet.
- Tense the muscles in that group, holding the tension for a few seconds.
- Release the tension and let the muscles completely relax.
- Pay attention to the sensation of relaxation in the muscles.
- Move on to the next muscle group, progressively working your way through the body, from head to toe.

- Repeat the process for each muscle group, allowing yourself to deeply relax.

Progressive muscle relaxation helps increase body awareness and promote relaxation by consciously releasing muscle tension. It can be particularly beneficial for reducing physical symptoms of stress, such as muscle tension, headaches, and bodily discomfort.

Both deep breathing and progressive muscle relaxation can be practiced individually or combined to enhance their relaxation effects. They are simple techniques that can be easily learned and incorporated into daily life to manage stress and promote overall well-being.

CHAPTER 6

6.1 Establishing Structure and Organization

Establishing structure and organization is an important aspect of overcoming OCD and maintaining a balanced life. When dealing with OCD, having a structured routine and organized approach can help reduce anxiety, manage symptoms, and improve overall well-being. Here are some strategies to establish structure and organization:

1. Set Clear Goals: Define clear goals and priorities for yourself. Identify what you want to achieve and what areas of your life require structure and organization. This could include daily routines, work or school tasks, personal projects, self-care, and leisure activities.

2. Create a Daily Schedule: Establish a daily schedule that includes specific time slots for different activities. Allocate dedicated time for work, chores, relaxation, exercise,

hobbies, and socializing. Having a structured routine can provide a sense of stability and reduce the feeling of being overwhelmed.

3. Use Planners or Calendars: Utilize planners, calendars, or digital tools to organize your tasks, appointments, and commitments. Write down important deadlines, events, and to-do lists. Break down large tasks into smaller, manageable steps and assign specific time slots to work on them.

4. Prioritize and Delegate: Learn to prioritize tasks based on their importance and urgency. Focus on completing high-priority tasks first before moving on to less urgent ones. Delegate responsibilities when possible and seek support from others, whether it's at work, home, or within your support network.

5. Declutter and Organize: Organize your physical space to reduce clutter and create a more calming environment. Clean and declutter your living or working area regularly. Find a specific place for your belongings and use storage solutions to keep things organized. A tidy space can contribute to a clearer mind and better focus.

6. Break Tasks into Manageable Chunks: If you find yourself getting overwhelmed by large tasks or projects, break them down into smaller, more manageable chunks. Focus on one task at a time and avoid multitasking, as it can increase stress and reduce efficiency.

7. Practice Time Management Techniques: Learn and implement time management techniques, such as the Pomodoro Technique or time-blocking. These techniques can help improve productivity by breaking your time into intervals and

allowing for focused work and regular breaks.

8. Establish Self-Care Routines: Incorporate self-care activities into your daily routine. This could include exercise, mindfulness or meditation practice, hobbies, relaxation techniques, or spending time with loved ones. Prioritizing self-care contributes to overall well-being and helps manage stress.

Remember that establishing structure and organization is a gradual process. Start with small steps and be flexible in adapting your routines as needed. It can be helpful to seek support from a therapist or counselor who can provide guidance and assistance in developing personalized strategies for managing OCD and maintaining a balanced life.

6.2 Prioritizing Self-Care

Prioritizing self-care is essential for maintaining balance, managing stress, and promoting overall well-being. Here are some key aspects to consider when prioritizing self-care:

1. Identify Your Needs: Take time to reflect on your physical, emotional, and mental well-being. Consider what activities or practices make you feel rejuvenated, relaxed, or fulfilled. It could be exercise, spending time in nature, engaging in creative hobbies, practicing mindfulness, or connecting with loved ones. Understanding your needs will help you prioritize self-care activities that truly resonate with you.

2. Make Self-Care a Priority: Recognize that self-care is not selfish but necessary for your overall well-being. Prioritize self-care by allocating dedicated time for it in your schedule. Treat it as an important appointment with yourself and commit to it as you would with any other commitment.

3. Set Boundaries: Establishing boundaries is crucial for protecting your time and energy. Learn to say no to activities or requests that don't align with your priorities or deplete your resources. Setting boundaries allows you to create space for self-care activities without feeling overwhelmed or overcommitted.

4. Practice Self-Compassion: Be kind and compassionate toward yourself. Acknowledge that self-care is a vital aspect of maintaining balance and managing stress. Let go of any guilt or self-judgment associated with taking time for yourself. Embrace the understanding that taking care of your needs enables you to show up fully for others.

5. Engage in Activities That Nourish You: Engage in activities that bring you joy, relaxation, or fulfillment. This could include engaging in physical exercise, practicing meditation or mindfulness, journaling,

reading, engaging in creative pursuits, spending time in nature, or indulging in a hobby you enjoy. Choose activities that resonate with you and help you recharge.

6. Prioritize Rest and Sleep: Rest and quality sleep are crucial for replenishing your energy and supporting overall well-being. Establish a consistent sleep routine that allows for sufficient rest. Prioritize relaxation activities before bedtime, such as reading a book, taking a warm bath, or practicing relaxation techniques, to promote better sleep.

7. Practice Mindfulness and Stress Reduction Techniques: Incorporate mindfulness and stress reduction techniques into your self-care routine. These practices, such as deep breathing exercises, meditation, yoga, or progressive muscle relaxation, can help calm your mind, reduce stress, and increase your overall sense of well-being.

8. Seek Support: Reach out for support from friends, family, or professionals when needed. Share your self-care goals and challenges with trusted individuals who can provide encouragement and accountability. Consider seeking guidance from a therapist or counselor who can offer specific strategies tailored to your needs.

Remember, self-care is an ongoing practice that requires attention and commitment. By prioritizing self-care, you not only benefit yourself but also enhance your ability to show up fully in other areas of your life, including relationships, work, and personal pursuits.

6.3. Healthy sleep habits

Developing healthy sleep habits, also known as sleep hygiene, is crucial for getting quality sleep and maintaining overall well-being. Here are some tips for cultivating healthy sleep habits:

1. Stick to a Consistent Sleep Schedule:
Establish a regular sleep schedule by going
to bed and waking up at the same time every
day, even on weekends. This helps regulate
your body's internal clock and promotes
better sleep quality.

2. Create a Restful Sleep Environment:
Make your sleep environment conducive to
sleep. Ensure your bedroom is cool, dark,
and quiet. Use comfortable bedding and
invest in a supportive mattress and pillows.
Consider using earplugs, eye masks, or
white noise machines if needed.

3. Limit Exposure to Electronics Before Bed:
The blue light emitted by electronic devices
like smartphones, tablets, and computers
can interfere with your sleep. Avoid using
these devices for at least an hour before bed.
Instead, engage in relaxing activities such as
reading a book or practicing relaxation
techniques.

4. Establish a Bedtime Routine: Develop a calming bedtime routine to signal to your body that it's time to wind down and prepare for sleep. This may include activities like taking a warm bath, practicing gentle stretching or yoga, listening to soft music, or engaging in a relaxation exercise.

5. Avoid Stimulants and Heavy Meals: Limit or avoid consuming caffeine, nicotine, and alcohol, particularly close to bedtime. These substances can disrupt your sleep patterns and prevent you from falling asleep or achieving restful sleep. Additionally, avoid heavy meals or large amounts of liquids close to bedtime to minimize discomfort and the need for nighttime bathroom trips.

6. Engage in Regular Exercise: Regular physical activity can contribute to better sleep. Engage in moderate exercise, such as walking, jogging, or cycling, during the day. However, avoid intense workouts close to

bedtime as they may increase alertness and make it harder to fall asleep.

7. Manage Stress and Relaxation: High levels of stress and anxiety can negatively impact sleep. Practice stress management techniques, such as mindfulness, deep breathing exercises, or meditation, to help calm your mind and promote relaxation before bed.

8. Avoid Napping or Keep It Short: If you struggle with nighttime sleep, limit daytime napping or keep it to short power naps of around 20 minutes. Longer or late afternoon naps can disrupt your sleep schedule and make it harder to fall asleep at night.

9. Monitor Your Sleep Environment: Pay attention to factors that may affect your sleep quality, such as excessive noise, uncomfortable room temperature, or an uncomfortable mattress. Make necessary

adjustments to optimize your sleep
environment for restful sleep.

10. Seek Professional Help if Needed: If you
consistently have trouble sleeping despite
practicing good sleep hygiene, consider
seeking guidance from a healthcare
professional or sleep specialist. They can
assess and address any underlying sleep
disorders or provide additional strategies to
improve your sleep.

Remember, developing healthy sleep habits
takes time and consistency. By prioritizing
sleep and implementing these strategies,
you can improve the quality and duration of
your sleep, leading to increased energy,
mental clarity, and overall well-being.

CHAPTER 7

7.1 Stress-Reduction Techniques

Stress-reduction techniques are valuable tools for managing and reducing stress levels, promoting relaxation, and enhancing overall well-being. Here are some effective stress-reduction techniques you can incorporate into your daily routine:

1. Deep Breathing: Practice deep breathing exercises, such as diaphragmatic breathing or belly breathing, to activate the body's relaxation response. Take slow, deep breaths, allowing your abdomen to rise as you inhale and fall as you exhale. Deep breathing helps calm the nervous system and reduces stress.

2. Progressive Muscle Relaxation (PMR): PMR involves systematically tensing and then relaxing different muscle groups in the body. Starting from your toes and moving up to your head, tense each muscle group

for a few seconds, then release the tension
and allow the muscles to relax. This
technique helps release physical tension and
promotes a state of relaxation.

3. Mindfulness Meditation: Engage in
mindfulness meditation to cultivate
present-moment awareness and
non-judgmental acceptance. Find a quiet
space, focus on your breath, and observe
your thoughts and sensations without
judgment. Regular mindfulness practice can
reduce stress, enhance emotional
well-being, and improve overall resilience.

4. Exercise and Physical Activity: Engage in
regular physical activity to reduce stress and
promote the release of endorphins, which
are natural mood-boosting chemicals in the
brain. Find activities that you enjoy,
whether it's walking, jogging, yoga, dancing,
or any other form of exercise that gets your
body moving.

5. Nature and Outdoor Time: Spend time in nature and reap the benefits of its calming and restorative effects. Take walks in natural settings, spend time in parks or gardens, or simply sit outside and enjoy the fresh air. Connecting with nature can help reduce stress and increase a sense of tranquility.

6. Journaling: Write down your thoughts, feelings, and concerns in a journal. This practice can help you process emotions, gain clarity, and release stress. Consider writing about gratitude, positive experiences, or exploring solutions to challenges you may be facing.

7. Engaging Hobbies: Participate in activities or hobbies that bring you joy and provide a sense of relaxation. It could be painting, playing a musical instrument, gardening, knitting, or any other activity that allows you to engage in a state of flow

and experience a sense of accomplishment and relaxation.

8. Social Support: Connect with loved ones, friends, or support groups. Sharing your feelings, thoughts, and experiences with trusted individuals can provide emotional support and help reduce stress. Whether it's through conversations, spending time together, or seeking advice, social support can help alleviate stress.

9. Time Management: Improve your time management skills to reduce stress and increase productivity. Prioritize tasks, break them down into manageable steps, and create a schedule that allows for breaks and self-care. Avoid overcommitting and learn to delegate or say no when necessary.

10. Relaxation Techniques: Explore other relaxation techniques such as listening to calming music, taking warm baths, practicing aromatherapy, using guided

imagery or visualization, or engaging in activities like coloring or puzzles that help redirect your focus and induce a state of relaxation.

Remember that everyone is unique, so experiment with different stress-reduction techniques to find what works best for you. Consider integrating these techniques into your daily routine and practice them consistently to experience their full benefits in managing stress and promoting overall well-being.

7.2 Anxiety Management Strategies

Managing anxiety is important for maintaining a sense of well-being and reducing the impact of anxiety on daily life. Here are some strategies to help manage anxiety:

1. Identify Triggers: Pay attention to situations, thoughts, or events that tend to trigger your anxiety. By identifying your

triggers, you can develop strategies to address them proactively.

2. Deep Breathing: Practice deep breathing exercises to help calm your nervous system and reduce anxiety. Take slow, deep breaths, focusing on your breath as it moves in and out of your body. This technique can help bring a sense of relaxation and grounding.

3. Challenge Negative Thoughts: When you notice negative or anxious thoughts, challenge their validity. Ask yourself if there is evidence to support these thoughts and consider alternative, more balanced perspectives. Reframing negative thoughts can help reduce anxiety.

4. Mindfulness and Meditation: Engage in mindfulness practices to cultivate present-moment awareness and reduce anxiety. Practice mindfulness meditation, body scans, or mindful walking to bring

your attention to the present and let go of anxious thoughts.

5. Physical Exercise: Regular physical activity can help reduce anxiety by releasing endorphins, improving mood, and providing a distraction from anxious thoughts. Find activities you enjoy and incorporate them into your routine.

6. Relaxation Techniques: Explore relaxation techniques such as progressive muscle relaxation, guided imagery, or visualization. These techniques help activate the body's relaxation response and reduce anxiety.

7. Self-Care: Prioritize self-care activities that promote relaxation and well-being. Engage in activities you enjoy, practice good sleep hygiene, maintain a healthy diet, and make time for hobbies, social connections, and relaxation.

8. Time Management: Poor time management can contribute to anxiety. Organize your time effectively by setting priorities, breaking tasks into manageable steps, and establishing realistic deadlines. This can help reduce feelings of overwhelm and create a sense of control.

9. Limit Stressful Stimuli: Minimize exposure to stressful stimuli when possible. This may involve setting boundaries with people or situations that trigger your anxiety, reducing exposure to news or social media, or creating a calm and clutter-free environment.

10. Seek Support: Reach out for support from friends, family, or mental health professionals. Talk about your feelings and concerns with trusted individuals who can provide understanding and guidance. Consider therapy or counseling to learn additional coping strategies and techniques.

Remember that managing anxiety is a personal journey, and it may take time to find the strategies that work best for you. Be patient and kind to yourself as you explore different techniques and make self-care a priority. If your anxiety persists or significantly interferes with your daily life, consider seeking professional help for a comprehensive evaluation and tailored treatment plan.

7.3 Coping with Uncertainty

Coping with uncertainty can be challenging, but there are strategies that can help you navigate through uncertain times more effectively. Here are some coping strategies for dealing with uncertainty:

1. Accept the Uncertainty: Acknowledge that uncertainty is a natural part of life and that it is not always possible to have complete control or predictability. Embrace the idea that uncertainty can offer opportunities for growth, learning, and adaptability.

2. Focus on What You Can Control: Shift your focus to aspects of the situation that you have control over. Identify the actions you can take or the decisions you can make in the present moment. By directing your energy towards what you can control, you can regain a sense of empowerment and reduce anxiety.

3. Practice Mindfulness: Engage in mindfulness techniques to stay grounded in the present moment. Instead of dwelling on the uncertainties of the future, focus on what is happening right now. Mindfulness helps cultivate acceptance, non-judgment, and resilience in the face of uncertainty.

4. Limit Exposure to Stressful Information: Limit your exposure to news or information that may increase your stress or anxiety. Constantly consuming distressing news or speculation about the future can intensify feelings of uncertainty. Stay informed, but

set boundaries to protect your mental well-being.

5. Maintain a Routine: Establish and maintain a daily routine as much as possible. Having structure and consistency in your day can provide a sense of stability and control amidst uncertainty. Prioritize self-care activities, work or study routines, and time for relaxation.

6. Practice Self-Care: Take care of your physical, emotional, and mental well-being. Engage in activities that help you relax and recharge, such as exercise, hobbies, meditation, or spending time in nature. Prioritize self-care practices that nourish and support your overall well-being.

7. Seek Social Support: Connect with others and seek support from friends, family, or support groups. Sharing your concerns, fears, and uncertainties with trusted individuals can provide comfort and

perspective. Engaging in meaningful connections can help reduce feelings of isolation and increase resilience.

8. Focus on the Present: Instead of getting caught up in future what-ifs, focus on the present moment and take things one step at a time. Break down tasks or challenges into smaller, manageable parts. By focusing on what needs to be done in the present, you can reduce overwhelm and anxiety.

9. Cultivate Resilience: Build resilience by adopting a growth mindset and reframing challenges as opportunities for personal growth and learning. Embrace uncertainty as a chance to develop adaptability, problem-solving skills, and resilience in the face of adversity.

10. Seek Professional Help if Needed: If uncertainty significantly impacts your well-being or daily functioning, consider seeking support from a mental health

professional. They can provide guidance, coping strategies, and tools to help you navigate through uncertainty more effectively.

Remember that coping with uncertainty is an ongoing process, and different strategies may work better for different individuals. Be patient with yourself and allow yourself to adapt to new circumstances. With time and practice, you can develop resilience and find ways to cope with uncertainty more effectively.

CHAPTER 8

8.1 Communicating with Loved Ones

Effective communication with loved ones is crucial for maintaining healthy relationships and navigating challenges together. Here are some tips for enhancing communication with your loved ones:

1. Active Listening: Practice active listening by giving your full attention to the person speaking. Maintain eye contact, avoid interrupting, and show genuine interest in what they are saying. Reflect back their thoughts and feelings to ensure understanding.

2. Express Empathy: Try to understand and empathize with the emotions and experiences of your loved ones. Validate their feelings and let them know that you are there to support them. Avoid judgment or minimizing their emotions.

3. Use "I" Statements: When expressing your own thoughts or concerns, use "I" statements to communicate your feelings and needs. This helps avoid blaming or accusing the other person, creating a more open and non-defensive atmosphere for discussion.

4. Be Mindful of Non-Verbal Communication: Non-verbal cues, such as facial expressions, body language, and tone of voice, can significantly impact communication. Be aware of your own non-verbal cues and pay attention to the non-verbal cues of your loved ones. They can convey emotions and provide additional context to the conversation.

5. Be Respectful and Constructive: Maintain a respectful and constructive tone during conversations. Avoid personal attacks, criticism, or defensiveness. Instead, focus on expressing your thoughts and feelings in

a way that promotes understanding and problem-solving.

6. Seek to Understand: Ask open-ended questions and seek clarification to better understand the perspectives and experiences of your loved ones. Show genuine curiosity and interest in their thoughts and feelings. This fosters deeper connection and can lead to more meaningful conversations.

7. Avoid Assumptions: Avoid making assumptions about what your loved ones are thinking or feeling. Instead, ask for clarification and encourage them to express themselves openly. This helps prevent misunderstandings and promotes effective communication.

8. Practice Conflict Resolution: In times of conflict, approach the situation with a mindset of finding a resolution rather than "winning" an argument. Use active listening,

express your concerns calmly, and work together to find mutually acceptable solutions. Compromise and find common ground whenever possible.

9. Timing and Environment: Choose an appropriate time and setting for important conversations. Find a quiet and comfortable space where both parties can focus without distractions. Timing is also crucial; avoid discussing sensitive or complex topics when either party is stressed, tired, or busy.

10. Practice Openness and Vulnerability: Foster an environment of trust and openness by being willing to share your thoughts, emotions, and vulnerabilities. This encourages your loved ones to do the same, fostering deeper connections and understanding.

Remember that effective communication is a continuous process that requires practice, patience, and mutual effort. By actively listening, expressing empathy, and creating a respectful and open atmosphere, you can strengthen your relationships and navigate challenges together with greater understanding and support.

8.2 Building a Support Network

Building a support network is crucial for your well-being and can provide you with emotional support, practical assistance, and a sense of belonging. Here are some steps to help you build a strong support network:

1. Identify Your Needs: Reflect on the types of support you need in your life. Consider emotional support, practical help, professional guidance, or specific interests or hobbies you'd like to pursue. Identifying your needs will help you seek out individuals or groups that can provide the support you require.

2. Reach Out to Trusted Individuals: Start by reaching out to family members, close

friends, or people you trust. Share your thoughts and feelings with them, and let them know that you value their support. Cultivate deeper connections by investing time and effort into these relationships.

3. Join Support Groups: Consider joining support groups or organizations that cater to your specific needs or interests. This could be local community groups, online forums, or social media communities. Engaging with individuals who share similar experiences can provide a sense of understanding, validation, and support.

4. Seek Professional Help: If you're dealing with specific challenges or mental health issues, consider seeking support from mental health professionals. Therapists, counselors, or support groups led by professionals can offer specialized guidance and strategies to help you cope and thrive.

5. Volunteer or Get Involved: Engage in volunteer work or community activities aligned with your interests and values. By contributing to a cause or organization, you can meet like-minded individuals and build connections based on shared passions. It's a way to give back while also building your support network.

6. Attend Workshops or Classes: Explore workshops, seminars, or classes related to your interests or personal development. This allows you to connect with individuals who share similar goals or passions. It can also provide opportunities for learning, growth, and networking.

7. Use Online Platforms: Utilize online platforms and social media networks to connect with individuals who share similar interests or experiences. Participate in online communities, forums, or groups where you can engage in discussions, seek advice, and offer support.

8. Be a Supportive Friend: Building a support network is a two-way street. Be supportive, empathetic, and available for others in your network. By being a good friend and providing support to others, you can create reciprocal relationships and strengthen your own support system.

9. Nurture Relationships: Regularly invest time and effort in maintaining your relationships. Reach out to your support network, schedule regular catch-ups, and engage in activities together. Openly communicate your appreciation for their support, and be available to listen and provide assistance when needed.

10. Be Patient: Building a support network takes time, so be patient and persistent. It's normal to experience ups and downs along the way. Focus on quality over quantity, and nurture the connections that bring you genuine support and positivity.

Remember that a support network is not just about receiving support but also about offering support to others. By building a strong network of caring and reliable individuals, you can enhance your well-being, navigate challenges more effectively, and experience a sense of belonging and connection.

8.3 Balancing Independence and Interdependence

Balancing independence and interdependence is about finding a healthy middle ground between autonomy and reliance on others. Here are some tips to help you achieve this balance:

1. Reflect on Your Needs: Understand your own needs for independence and interdependence. Consider the areas where you prefer to be self-reliant and those where you benefit from support or collaboration

with others. This self-awareness will guide you in finding the right balance.

2. Cultivate Self-Reliance: Foster a sense of independence by developing your skills, knowledge, and capabilities. Take responsibility for your own well-being and strive for personal growth. Build confidence in your ability to handle various aspects of life on your own.

3. Practice Effective Communication: Clearly communicate your boundaries, preferences, and needs to others. Be open about what you can handle independently and when you require assistance. Effective communication ensures that both you and those around you understand your expectations and can respect your boundaries.

4. Seek Support When Needed: Recognize that it is okay to ask for help when you need it. Interdependence involves reaching out to

others and leveraging their skills, expertise, and support when necessary. Don't hesitate to seek assistance from your support network or professionals in areas where you need guidance or support.

5. Foster Collaboration: Embrace collaboration and teamwork in areas where it enhances your growth and effectiveness. Recognize that working with others can bring fresh perspectives, new ideas, and shared success. Be open to learning from others and contributing to joint efforts.

6. Set Healthy Boundaries: Establish boundaries to maintain a healthy balance between independence and interdependence. Clearly define what you are comfortable with and communicate it to others. Be assertive in saying no when necessary and prioritize your own well-being.

7. Embrace Interconnectedness: Recognize that human beings are inherently interconnected and that healthy relationships are vital to our well-being. Embrace the support, love, and connections that others offer. Allow yourself to lean on others during challenging times and reciprocate by being supportive when they need it.

8. Regular Self-Reflection: Regularly reflect on your level of independence and interdependence. Assess whether you have been leaning too heavily on others or neglecting your own independence. Adjust and calibration is needed to maintain a healthy balance.

9. Practice Self-Care: Prioritize self-care activities that nurture your independence and well-being. Engage in hobbies, self-reflection, and personal growth initiatives that foster your individuality. Taking care of yourself allows you to bring

your best self to relationships and collaborations.

10. Embrace Flexibility: Recognize that the balance between independence and interdependence may shift depending on life circumstances. Be flexible and adaptable, adjusting your approach as needed to find the optimal balance at different stages of your life.

Remember, finding the right balance between independence and interdependence is a personal journey. It may vary for different individuals and situations. Regular self-reflection, effective communication, and a willingness to adapt will help you navigate this balance and lead a fulfilling and connected life.

CHAPTER 9

9.1 Relapse Prevention Strategies

Relapse prevention strategies are essential for maintaining progress and preventing setbacks in overcoming OCD. Here are some strategies to help you prevent relapse:

1. Continuing Treatment: Stay engaged in your treatment plan, whether it's therapy, medication, or a combination of both. Regularly attend therapy sessions and follow your prescribed medication regimen as advised by your healthcare provider. Consistency in treatment is crucial for long-term management of OCD.

2. Identify Triggers: Recognize the specific triggers or situations that can lead to OCD symptoms resurfacing. It could be certain environments, stressors, or thoughts that exacerbate your OCD. Identify these triggers and develop strategies to manage them effectively.

3. Develop Coping Skills: Learn and practice coping skills that help you manage OCD symptoms when they arise. This may include relaxation techniques, mindfulness, deep breathing exercises, or engaging in activities that provide a sense of calm and distraction. Having a toolbox of coping skills can empower you to respond to triggers in a healthy way.

4. Challenge Negative Thoughts: OCD is often fueled by negative and intrusive thoughts. Practice cognitive restructuring techniques to challenge and reframe these thoughts. Replace irrational or obsessive thoughts with more realistic and balanced ones. This can help reduce anxiety and prevent the escalation of OCD symptoms.

5. Maintain a Support Network: Surround yourself with a supportive network of family, friends, or support groups who understand your challenges and provide

encouragement. Lean on them during difficult times, and don't hesitate to reach out for support when needed.

6. Engage in Self-Care: Prioritize self-care activities that promote your overall well-being. Take care of your physical health through regular exercise, a balanced diet, and adequate sleep. Attend to your emotional needs by engaging in activities you enjoy, practicing relaxation techniques, and managing stress effectively.

7. Set Realistic Goals: Set realistic and achievable goals for yourself. Break down large goals into smaller, manageable steps. Celebrate your progress along the way to boost motivation and confidence.

8. Monitor Your Progress: Keep track of your progress in managing OCD symptoms. Regularly monitor your thoughts, behaviors, and triggers to identify patterns or warning signs of relapse. This self-awareness will

help you take proactive steps to address symptoms before they worsen.

9. Develop a Relapse Prevention Plan: Work with your mental health professional to create a relapse prevention plan. This plan should include specific strategies and actions to take if you notice a recurrence of OCD symptoms. Having a plan in place can help you respond effectively and minimize the impact of a potential relapse.

10. Practice Self-Compassion: Be kind and compassionate towards yourself throughout your recovery journey. Remember that setbacks are a normal part of the process, and relapse does not mean failure. Treat yourself with understanding and patience, and seek help and support when needed.

Remember, relapse prevention is an ongoing process, and strategies may need to be adjusted over time. Stay proactive, maintain healthy habits, and seek professional guidance when necessary to effectively manage and prevent relapse in your journey towards overcoming OCD.

9.2 Self-Reflection and Self-Care Practices

Self-reflection and self-care practices are essential for maintaining balance, promoting well-being, and nurturing personal growth. Here are some self-reflection and self-care practices you can incorporate into your life:

1. Journaling: Set aside time for journaling to explore your thoughts, emotions, and experiences. Write freely and honestly, allowing yourself to gain insights, process feelings, and gain a deeper understanding of yourself.

2. Mindfulness Meditation: Practice mindfulness meditation to cultivate present-moment awareness and non-judgmental acceptance. Set aside dedicated time each day to focus on your

breath, sensations, and thoughts. This practice can help reduce stress, increase self-awareness, and enhance overall well-being.

3. Gratitude Practice: Regularly express gratitude for the positive aspects of your life. Take time to reflect on the things you appreciate and write them down or share them with others. Gratitude practice can shift your focus towards positivity and enhance your overall sense of well-being.

4. Self-Compassion: Be kind and compassionate towards yourself. Treat yourself with the same empathy and understanding you would offer to a close friend. Practice self-compassion by acknowledging your struggles, forgiving yourself for mistakes, and embracing your imperfections.

5. Setting Boundaries: Reflect on your boundaries and ensure they align with your

needs and values. Identify areas where you may need to set clear boundaries in relationships, work, or other areas of your life. Setting and maintaining healthy boundaries is crucial for self-care and maintaining a sense of balance.

6. Disconnecting from Technology: Take intentional breaks from technology to recharge and reconnect with yourself. Disconnecting from constant notifications and distractions allows you to be present in the moment and engage in activities that promote self-care, such as reading, walking in nature, or spending quality time with loved ones.

7. Engaging in Creative Activities: Explore creative outlets that bring you joy and allow for self-expression. This can include activities such as painting, writing, playing a musical instrument, or engaging in crafts. Engaging in creative endeavors fosters

self-discovery, relaxation, and a sense of fulfillment.

8. Practicing Self-Care Rituals: Incorporate regular self-care rituals into your routine. This could be taking a warm bath, practicing a skincare routine, indulging in a hobby you enjoy, or setting aside time for activities that recharge and rejuvenate you. Prioritize self-care as a non-negotiable part of your daily or weekly routine.

9. Reflecting on Personal Values and Goals: Take time to reflect on your personal values and long-term goals. Evaluate whether your current actions align with these values and goals. Make any necessary adjustments to ensure you are living a life that is authentic and meaningful to you.

10. Seeking Support: Reach out for support when needed. This could involve confiding in a trusted friend, family member, or seeking professional help from a therapist or

counselor. Don't hesitate to seek assistance and guidance when navigating challenges or when you feel overwhelmed.

Remember, self-reflection and self-care practices are unique to each individual. Find what resonates with you and make these practices a priority in your life. Regular self-reflection and self-care allow you to nurture your well-being, maintain balance, and cultivate a deeper understanding of yourself.

9.3 Continuing Professional Support

Continuing professional support is crucial for ongoing growth, development, and well-being. Here are some reasons why it is important to continue professional support:

1. Maintenance of Progress: Professional support, such as therapy or counseling, provides ongoing guidance and assistance in managing challenges and maintaining

progress. It allows you to address any emerging issues, reinforce coping skills, and navigate new situations or triggers that may arise.

2. Accountability and Motivation: Regular sessions with a mental health professional help you stay accountable to your goals and provide motivation to continue working towards them. The support and encouragement from a professional can be instrumental in overcoming obstacles and staying committed to your well-being.

3. Deeper Self-Understanding: Continued professional support allows for deeper self-exploration and understanding. Through ongoing discussions and insights gained from therapy, you can uncover patterns, underlying beliefs, and unresolved issues that may impact your well-being. This self-awareness is essential for personal growth and making positive changes in your life.

4. Skill Building and Coping Strategies: Professionals can help you develop and refine coping strategies tailored to your specific needs. They can teach you new skills, such as stress management techniques, communication skills, or problem-solving strategies, that can enhance your ability to navigate challenges effectively.

5. Addressing Relapses or Setbacks: If you experience a relapse or setback in your progress, professional support is invaluable in helping you address and overcome it. Therapists or counselors can provide the necessary guidance, tools, and support to get back on track and prevent further setbacks.

6. Mental Health Maintenance: Just as you take care of your physical health through regular check-ups, professional support ensures the maintenance of your mental

health. Regular sessions can serve as a proactive measure to monitor your well-being, identify potential issues early on, and prevent the escalation of mental health challenges.

7. Support During Life Transitions: Life transitions, such as career changes, relationship changes, or significant life events, can be stressful and impact your mental health. Professional support during these periods can provide valuable guidance, perspective, and coping strategies to navigate these transitions successfully.

8. Integration of New Skills: As you acquire new skills and strategies through therapy or counseling, professional support helps you integrate these tools into your daily life. Professionals can provide guidance on how to apply what you've learned in therapy to real-world situations and support you in practicing and reinforcing these skills.

9. Validation and Empathy: Professional support offers a safe and non-judgmental space where you can express your thoughts, feelings, and experiences. The validation and empathy provided by a mental health professional can be validating and therapeutic, helping you process emotions, gain clarity, and feel understood.

10. Prevention of Relapse: Professional support can play a vital role in preventing relapse by addressing underlying issues, reinforcing coping mechanisms, and providing ongoing support. By continuing professional support, you can reduce the risk of regression and maintain a higher level of overall well-being.

Remember, the duration and frequency of professional support may vary depending on

Conclusion

In conclusion, overcoming OCD and achieving a life of balance requires a multifaceted approach that includes various strategies and interventions. This book has explored the different aspects of OCD, including its causes, symptoms, impact on daily life, and the role of mental health professionals in diagnosis and treatment. We have delved into different treatment options, such as therapy and medication, and explored specific techniques like Cognitive Behavioral Therapy (CBT), Exposure and Response Prevention (ERP), and mindfulness-based practices.

Additionally, we have discussed the importance of self-reflection and self-care practices in maintaining well-being, managing stress, and preventing relapse. Strategies for establishing structure and organization, prioritizing self-care, promoting healthy sleep habits, and managing anxiety and uncertainty have been highlighted. Furthermore, we have emphasized the significance of building a support network, effective communication, and balancing independence with interdependence in fostering a balanced life.

Lastly, we have touched upon relapse prevention strategies and the importance of continuing professional support to sustain progress, address setbacks, and nurture personal growth. By integrating these strategies and practices into your life, you can overcome OCD and cultivate a sense of balance, well-being, and fulfillment.

Remember, everyone's journey is unique, and it's important to consult with mental health professionals for personalized guidance and support. With determination, self-compassion, and the tools provided in this book, you can embark on a path towards overcoming OCD and living a life of balance.

www.ingramcontent.com/pod-product-compliance
Lightning Source LLC
Chambersburg PA
CBHW060112260726
48658CB00004B/1512